WILDERNESS SELF RELIANCE

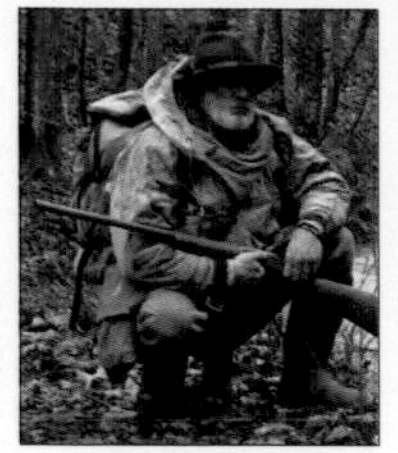

My Pathfinder Outdoor Survival Guides offer a simple and common sense approach to being prepared for any survival situation. If you practice the skills and techniques in this guide, you will be prepared when the occasion arises. Most important is that you develop the ability to adapt, improvise and overcome adversity by learning to use what is available to you. And that you stay firm in your belief that you CAN survive – never give up.

The Pathfinder School System®

Created as a teaching tool for my students in Wilderness Self Reliance, the Pathfinder School System represents the wisdom of the ancient scouts who ventured ahead of nomadic tribes to find fresh areas to support their community.

These "Pathfinders" had to accurately identify the perfect spot to sustain their tribes – they had to recognize the resources that would afford food, shelter, water, medicines and protection – the very same resources a person would need today. This system is designed to introduce you to the knowledge you need to increase your survivability.

Staying uninjured and healthy are critical factors to survival. Every person who spends time in the wilderness should have, at the very least, basic first aid training. With that, a positive attitude and some basic remedies should you become injured or ill, you have what it takes to survive.

People lost or stranded in wilderness situations often die of hypothermia (a drop in core body temperature), hyperthermia (a rise in core body temperature) and shock. Learn how to avoid these conditions and what to do if the situation occurs. Anticipate that you may experience an injury and have the basics in your survival kit that will help you administer self aid should the need arise.

Before You Go

Take first aid training. Nothing takes the place of first aid knowledge and professional medical help. In all cases you are advised to seek medical attention at the earliest possible time. This guide, however, is about survival situations when you are far away from civilization and the emergency resources we all rely on.

The remedies outlined in this guide are emergency survival strategies and should be used as a last resort when you have no other means of treating your injuries or illness.

Dave Canterbury is a master woodsman with over 20 years of experience working in many dangerous environments. He has taught survival and survival methods to hundreds of students and professionals in the US and around the world. His common sense approach to survivability is recognized as one of the most effective systems of teaching known today. For information on Pathfinder programs and materials visit http://www.thepathfinderschoolllc.com.

N.B. – The publisher makes no representation or warranties with respect to the accuracy, completeness, correctness or usefulness of this information and specifically disclaims any implied warranties of fitness for a particular purpose. The advice, strategies and/or techniques contained herein may not be suitable for all individuals. The publisher shall not be responsible for any physical harm (up to and including death), loss of profit or other commercial damage. The publisher assumes no liability brought or instituted by individuals or organizations arising out of or relating in any way to the application and/or use of the information, advice and strategies contained herein.

Waterford Press publishes reference guides that introduce readers to nature observation, outdoor recreation and survival skills. Product information is featured on the website: **www.waterfordpress.com**

Text & illustrations © 2012, 2023 Waterford Press Inc. All rights reserved. Images marked IC © Iris Canterbury 2012, 2023. Cover photo © Shutterstock. To order or for information on custom published products please call 800-434-2555 or emailorderdesk@waterfordpress.com. For permissions or to share comments emaileditor@waterfordpress.com. 2306505

$7.95 U.S.
$ 9.95 CAN

ISBN 978-1-58355-718-1
50795
9 781583 557181
UPC 8 84682 00512 2

10 9 8 7 6 5 4 3 2 1

Made in the USA

WILDERNESS FIRST AID – A Waterproof Folding Guide to Common Sense Self Care

PATHFINDER OUTDOOR SURVIVAL GUIDE™

WILDERNESS FIRST AID

A Waterproof Folding Guide to Common Sense Self Care

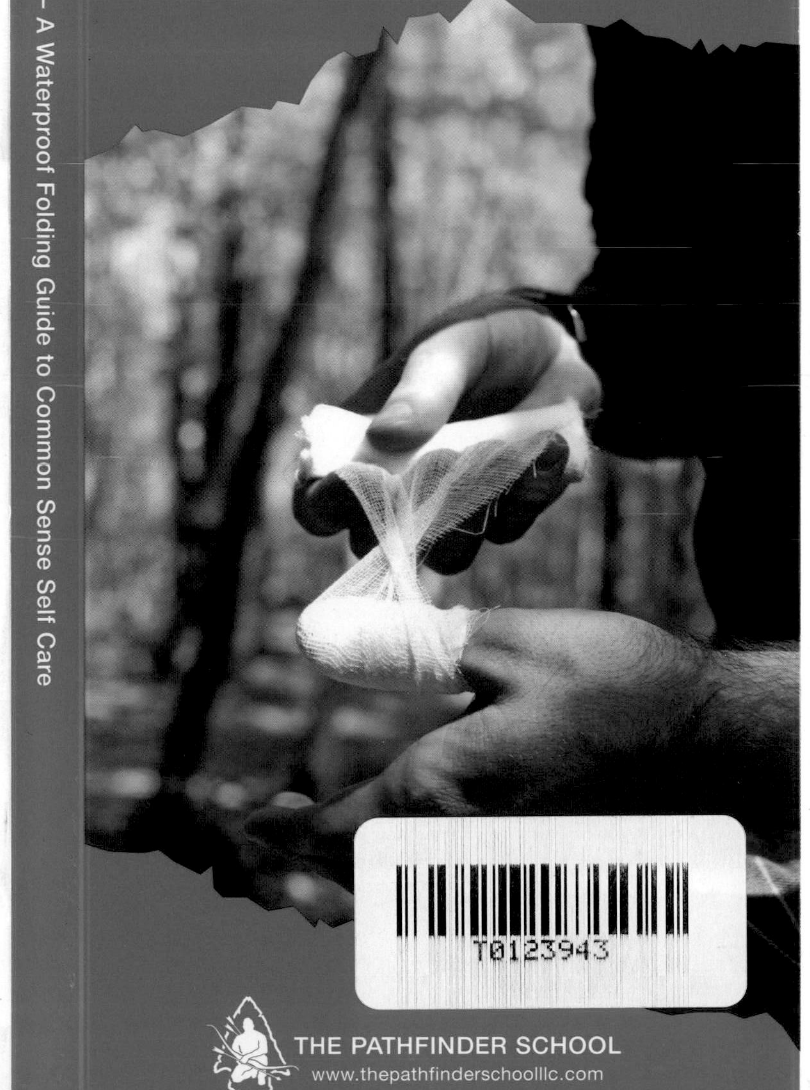

T0123943

THE PATHFINDER SCHOOL
www.thepathfinderschoolllc.com

STAY HEALTHY & UNINJURED

In survival situations, avoiding injury is paramount. In the same way that you calculate an energy expenditure versus the calorie gain when you are seeking food, you must look at the risk of injury as you consider activities and routes.

Stay healthy by maintaining good personal hygiene. Try to wash every day, especially your hands and body areas that could stay moist, harbor bugs, or form rashes and blisters.

If you have no soap, use sand or white ashes. Remove clothing where/when it makes sense to let the sun and fresh air get at your clothes and body. Clean your teeth with fibrous twigs or cattails. Most importantly, take good care of your feet. If you feel blisters or "hot" spots forming, stop to air out your shoes, try to refit your socks (dry them if wet) and use moss if available to cushion the wear spot. If a blister forms and bursts, treat it as you would an open wound.

Avoid injury by recognizing your limitations and the hazards in a particular environment. In extreme heat or cold, it is essential to preserve your core body temperature and avoid heat stroke or frostbite.

In mountainous terrain, in addition to exposure, risks include rock slides and falls. In wooded areas, especially in windy or storm conditions, people are injured by falling trees. Around lakes and rivers, hypothermia will result from immersion in water – a person can lose core body temperature even in waters as warm as 80° F (26.7 C) if they are immersed for an extended period of time. Desert, high altitude and arid conditions bring the risk of dehydration and hyper- or hypothermia. All environments include the hazards of animal stings or bites and strain or sprain injuries from a casual stumble or fall.

FIRST AID STRATEGY

Proficiency in emergency first aid can make the difference between life and death in a survival situation. Avoid panic and stay calm. Compose yourself and those who can help and take charge of the situation.

1. **Assess the Situation** – Are you or the victim in any danger? Make sure the area is safe before providing assistance or move to safety as possible. Only move victims when necessary.
2. **Immediately call 911 or send for medical help if possible.**
3. **Check pulse, airway and breathing quickly** (not more than 10 seconds).
4. **Respond to obvious bleeding and administer CPR to restore breathing and pulse.**

In all cases, the strategy is: remain safe; avoid compromising personal safety; stabilize victim until rescued and to the point suitable for transport to a medical treatment facility.

Always take precautions to avoid becoming contaminated by another person's body fluids.

VITAL SIGNS

- The normal range for vital signs varies with age, weight, gender and overall health.
- Adult heart rate ranges from 60 to 100 beats per minute.
- Adult respiratory rate ranges from 12 to 20 breaths per minute.
- Both heart rate and breathing rates are generally higher for children and infants.
- The other two vital signs, blood pressure and body temperature, are not easily measured without the proper equipment but should be monitored if possible.

PRIMARY RESPONSE

Assess the Victim's Condition

Check circulation, airway and breathing for no more than 10 seconds before you begin administering first aid; immediate action is required when those body functions are impaired. Respond to obvious bleeding and administer CPR to restore breathing and pulse.

Look for bleeding and check pulse by placing two fingers on the side of the windpipe nearest you, pressing lightly. For infants, check pulse on the inside of the upper arm between elbow and shoulder. If no pulse or breathing, begin CPR immediately.

Unconscious Victim Not Breathing

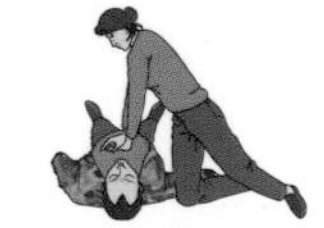

1. If face-down, roll the victim onto back while supporting the head, neck and back.
2. Check pulse for no longer than 10 seconds. If no pulse begin CPR.
3. Administer 30 hard-and-fast chest compressions at a rate of 100 to 120 compressions per minute.
4. Position head and open airway using jaw thrust method if you suspect spinal injury. Otherwise use head tilt/chin lift method.
5. Give two rescue breaths.
6. If air does not go in, retilt and try again.
7. Continue CPR alternating 30 compressions with two rescue breaths until breathing is restored or an advanced medical responder arrives to relieve you.

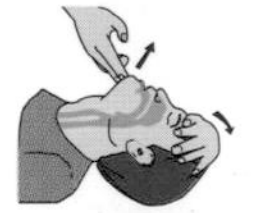

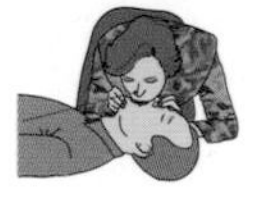

If uncomfortable with rescue breathing, perform continuous compressions at the same rate. Good compressions are the primary need in CPR.

Unconscious Victim Breathing

1. If breathing is detected but you cannot wake the victim, do not start CPR; continue to call for medical help.
2. If you suspect spinal injury, leave the victim on his/her back if possible.
3. If no spinal injury is suspected, move victim into recovery position.

Conscious Victim Breathing

If the victim is responsive and there is no severe life-threatening bleeding or injury:

1. Tell the victim your name, what your qualifications are (as in, "I have CPR training") and ask permission to provide care.
2. Ask where he/she hurts or feels differently. Evaluate breathing. If victim is talking, breathing is probably OK. If victim holds throat or responds in squeaking/wheezing noises, look for choking or chest wounds.
3. Check for shock, fractures, burns and other obvious injuries.
4. If no spinal injury is suspected, move victim into recovery position.

RECOVERY POSITION

If the victim is responsive, which implies consciousness and a pulse, and there is no evidence of severe injury or trauma to the head or spine, move victim into recovery position.

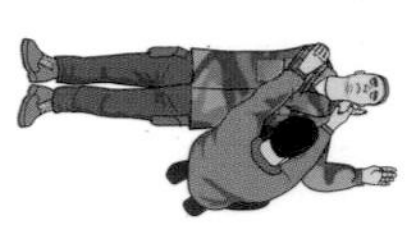

Carefully roll person onto his/her side.

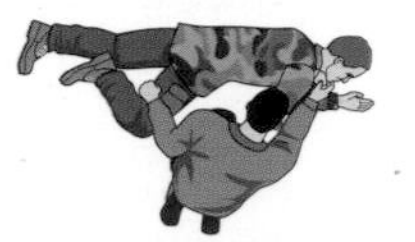

Bend arm and leg outward to stop victim from lying flat.

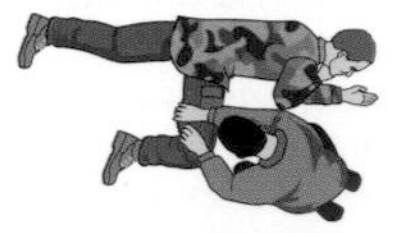

Extend head and tilt jaw forward to keep airway open.

CPR – CHEST COMPRESSIONS

The American Heart Association recommends a hand-only CPR for both untrained bystanders and for trained first responders that are not part of a response to the incident. The strength of the compressions differs from adults, children, infants and the elderly but the frequency and pace are the same. Compressions are delivered at a rate of 100 to 120 compressions a minute, allowing the chest to spring back after each push. Your knees should be near the person's body, spread about shoulder width apart for stability.

Adult & Juvenile

1. Place the heel of your hand on the center of the victim's chest, level with the nipple line. Take care to not press on the ribs of the soft upper abdomen. Cover your first hand with your second hand, interlock your fingers and lift them clear of the victim's chest.
2. Kneel with your shoulders over the breastbone and your arms straight. Press down "hard-and-fast," pushing at least 2 in. (5 cm) into the chest at a rate of 100 to 120 compressions per minute.
3. Continue chest compressions until there are signs of movement or until emergency responders arrive.

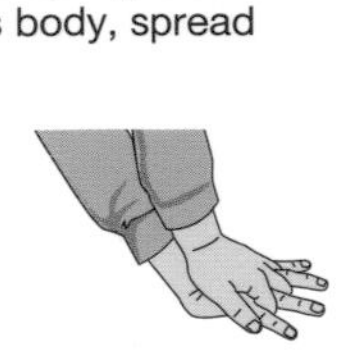

Press with heel of hand only, keeping fingers off chest.

Young Child (1-12 years old)

1. For children under 12 years old, use one hand only.
2. Compressions for children should only be about 1½ in. to 2 in. (4-5 cm); Treat fragile elderly as you would a child, as their bones can be brittle and easily fractured.

Infant (under 1 year old)

1. For infants, use two fingers.
2. Compressions for infants should be no more than 1½ in. (4 cm) deep.

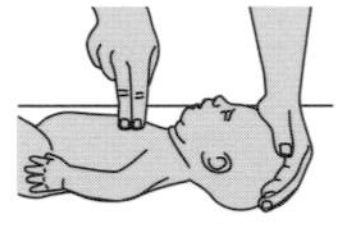

For infants, use two fingers only.

CPR – RESCUE BREATHING

The American Heart Association recommends rescue breathing with compressions in the event of drowning, opioid overdose, carbon monoxide poisoning and for unresponsive infants (caused by SIDS or suffocation). In those cases, and with the guidance of 911 dispatchers or trained first responders, these are key steps and techniques:

Clear the airway and position the head properly

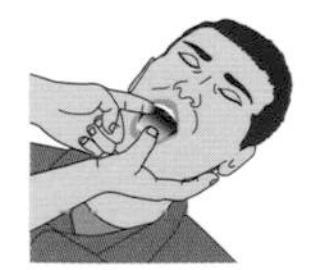

Clear any obstructions (food, tongue, false teeth, vomit, etc.) by looking inside the mouth and sweeping the object out with a finger. Position the victim's head to open the airway then check again for obstruction before beginning rescue breaths.

Head Tilt/Chin Lift Method (when no spinal injury suspected)

1. Kneel at the victim's shoulder.
2. Place one hand on victim's forehead and apply firm backward pressure to tilt head back.
3. Place fingertips of your other hand under the tip of the chin and bring the chin forward.

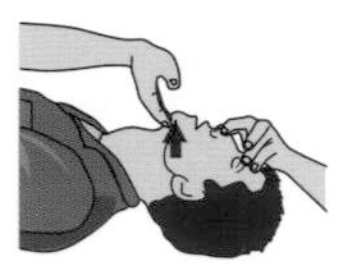

Lift chin forward until upper and lower teeth are almost together, but be sure mouth is not closed.

CPR – RESCUE BREATHING

Begin Rescue Breathing

A lack of breathing or pulse can be common signs of cardiac arrest. Noisy, gasping or irregular breathing and bluish lips indicate breathing distress. Be sure the victim is on a hard, flat surface.

Adult & Child

1. Place your hands in position; apply 30 chest compressions.
2. With the victim's head in position, pinch the nose shut. Take a normal breath in, seal your lips over the victim's mouth so air will not escape; blow until the chest rises (about 1 second per blow).
3. Administer breath until you see the chest rise, listen or feel for exhale, then quickly administer the second breath and listen/feel again.
4. If no breath, continue 30 chest compressions followed by 2 breaths sequence until breathing resumes or advanced medical help arrives.

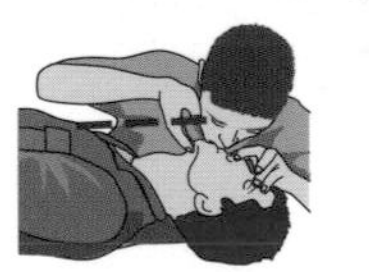

Infants

1. Place your hand in position (two fingers) at sternum.
2. Apply 30 gentle compressions (rate same as for adults).
3. Position victim's head. Place mouth over victim's mouth and nose and use small breaths (don't blow—just exhale into airways).
4. Watch for chest to rise. Do not overinflate. Repeat second breath.
5. If no breath, continue 30 chest compressions/2 breaths sequence until breathing resumes or advanced medical help arrives.

HEAD INJURY

Symptoms

Exposed skull; Slurred speech; Confused; Bleeding scalp; Unequal pupils, bruising behind eyes; Fluid draining from nose or ear; Nausea and/or vomiting; Convulsions; Yawning and sighing; Gradual loss of consciousness.

Action

1. Monitor for shock, bleeding and difficulty breathing every 10 minutes.
2. If the victim is convulsing, ease them to the ground in a safe area and support their head and neck; do not restrict limbs since this can lead to broken bones.
3. Find medical aid as quickly as possible.

HEAT EXPOSURE

Heatstroke (the most serious of all heat-related illnesses)

Heatstroke occurs when the victim's body temperature rises above 104°. It is a life-threatening emergency; the victim is overheating and must be cooled aggressively. Seek medical help immediately.

Heat Exhaustion (Hyperthermia)

In heat exhaustion, the victim is dehydrated, not overheated.

Symptoms

Shallow, rapid breathing; Weak rapid pulse; Chalky pallor; Excessive sweating; Headache or dizziness; Cramps; Spasms; Nausea and vomiting; Loss of consciousness (severe).

Action

1. Place victim in a cool area. Loosen clothing. Monitor breathing and be ready to administer CPR. If victim is breathing but unconscious, move to the recovery position.
2. Administer fluids if victim is awake and can swallow. A person who continues to sweat is likely in the first stage of heat exhaustion and can be given a decent amount of fluid orally. A person who has stopped sweating and is dry should be given very modest amounts of fluid and transported to a medical facility.

COLD EXPOSURE

Cold Exposure (Hypothermia)
Symptoms

Shivering; Slurred speech; Drowsiness; Loss of consciousness; Weak pulse; Shallow breathing; Low body temperature.

Action

1. Prevent further heat loss; move to sheltered area, remove any wet clothing and cover victim's head. Rewarm victim's body with blankets, campfire or the heat of another's body. **DO NOT place in hot water.**
2. Monitor breathing and be prepared to administer CPR. If victim is breathing but unconscious, move to the recovery position.
3. If condition does not improve, seek medical help. If moving the victim, transport them gently; rough handling can cause cardiac arrest (also see "Moving Injured Victim").

Frostbite
Symptoms

Flesh becoming white, waxy, numb and hard.

Action

1. Remove jewelry and restrictive clothing.
2. Rewarm affected area by placing it next to warm body parts.
3. Do not rub affected area or expose it to open fire.
4. If part is completely frozen, rewarm as soon as practical and only if you are able to keep the affected area warmed; immobilize and get medical assistance ASAP.

SHOCK

Shock occurs when the cardiovascular system cannot provide sufficient circulation to all parts of the body. Shock often follows severe injury or trauma and can usually be attributed to a drop in blood pressure due to severe internal or external bleeding, burns, crush injuries, severe allergic reactions and cardiovascular failure. Symptoms may be immediate or delayed.

Symptoms

Fast, shallow breathing; Weak and then rapid pulse; Chalky pallor; Cold, clammy skin; Thirst; Nausea and/or vomiting; Yawning and sighing; Gradual loss of consciousness.

Action

1. Lay victim on his/her back. Loosen any tight clothing, remove jewelry and cover with coat or poncho to help them maintain body heat. If victim is unconscious, turn their head to one side to prevent him from choking if they vomit.
2. Assess and manage any obvious injuries; note that there may be internal bleeding. Do not give liquids.
3. Keep victim calm, warm, comfortable and encouraged. Do not leave them alone unless necessary.
4. Monitor and record the victim's pulse and breathing until help arrives. Be prepared to resuscitate.

HEART ATTACK

Symptoms

Pale; Weak; Could be nauseated; May feel sharp or dull pain in chest radiating to shoulder, jaw or back.

Action

1. Have victim sit down to avoid exertion.
2. Seek medical help immediately.
3. Determine if victim has prescribed medicine, if so, encourage them to take it.
4. Administer 325mg (1 adult tablet or 4 baby tablets) of Aspirin orally and chewed.

BLEEDING

Symptoms

Injuries that cut an artery can be recognized by the bleeding that comes in strong spurts in time with the heartbeat (arterial bleeding). The more common injuries cut veins, causing blood to ooze from the wounded area. Both types of bleeding can be controlled by applying pressure to the wound site, then elevating the injured area above the level of the heart if possible.

Action

1. Check wound to ensure there are no embedded objects.
2. Apply clean dressing over the bleeding point and secure the dressing over the wound. If blood seeps through add a second dressing. If blood seeps through again, remove dressings and start again, ensuring that pressure is applied accurately over the wound.
3. Have victim lie down and watch for signs of shock. Raise and support the limb or injured area.
4. Check circulation (pulse) after bandaging or splinting. Always check both limbs simultaneously and compare pulse to make sure circulation is not obstructed.

Tourniquets

Any arterial bleeding on a limb or massive bleeding to a limb requires a tourniquet immediately. Use if a pressure dressing under a firm hand continues to soak with blood and the wound continues to bleed after 10 minutes.

1. To prepare a tourniquet, use a 6-8 in. (15-20 cm) piece of cloth or bandaging.
2. Wrap it around the limb placed 2-3 in. above the wound and not over a joint. Tie the ends of the cloth around a stick or other solid cylindrical object then twist the cloth in circles around the object until bleeding is slowed to a minimum.
3. Secure the object in place by tying or otherwise making it immobile so tension remains on the tourniquet.
4. If you are not accompanying the victim to the hospital, mark him/her with a "T" and the time (in his/her own blood if necessary) near the TQ site to indicate to emergency personnel that a tourniquet is applied.

EMBEDDED OBJECT

Action

1. Do not remove object; pinch edges of the wound together next to the object to control severe bleeding.
2. When bleeding subsides, drape cleanest available material over the wound and the embedded object.
3. Very carefully, build up padding using sphagnum moss or other soft clean material on either side of the object to keep it from moving. Build up padding until you can bandage the area above and below the object without putting pressure on it. Keep wounded area as still as possible during transport to a medical facility.

INFECTION

Always monitor wounds for signs of infection including increasing pain, redness and swelling, white pus, signs of red streaks under skin near wound and fever. If these signs worsen, seek medical help ASAP.

MOVING INJURED PERSONS

Do not attempt to move a victim until you assess his/her condition. If you suspect a spinal injury, do not move him/her unless situation is life-threatening; movement could cause paralysis or death.

Symptoms

Neck or back pain; Inability to move limbs or extremities; Numbness of limbs or extremities.

Action

1. If you suspect a spinal injury and have to move the victim, only do so if it is possible without moving or twisting head, neck or back.
2. Using several people, carefully immobilize victim's head, neck and back to prevent ANY movement.
3. DO NOT raise or twist head. Place heavy, padded objects on either side of the head or neck. Move victim on a rigid, flat surface.

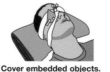

Note that up to 25% of victims paralyzed in accidents become paralyzed as a result of being moved improperly. The remedies outlined in this Guide are emergency survival strategies and should only be followed as a last resort when medical help is not available and you have no other means of treating your injuries or illness.

BURNS

Burns cause intense pain and fluid loss and are susceptible to infection. Severe burns can be fatal.

Symptoms

First-degree Burn – Redness and swelling of skin.

Second-degree Burn – Blistered skin in burn area, often accompanied by severe pain.

Third-degree Burn – Pale, charred skin; Nerves are often damaged so pain is less severe.

Action

1. Expose the burned area. Gently remove any burned clothing but DO NOT remove any clothing sticking to burn. Remove any jewelry or watches.
2. DO NOT touch or clean burned area, pop blisters or apply any ointments or sprays to the burn.
3. Flush burned area with cold water until pain eases.
4. Cover the wound with clean dry cloth (bandages) if possible. Place dressing directly over the wound, wind the tails in opposite directions and securely tie at the edge of the dressing. You do not want the dressing to slip. If a dressing is not available, cover the area with a clean cloth or plastic to prevent infection.
5. Monitor for shock and check vital signs every 10 minutes until help arrives. If the victim is not nauseous, give small amounts of water.

BLISTERS & RASHES

The best treatment for blisters and rashes is to avoid them. If you feel a hot spot forming on your foot, stop and take your shoes off, dry your socks and try to pad the area if you have to keep moving. Apply the padding in an area larger than the actual hotspot to protect it, DO NOT burst a blister unless you have alcohol and clean dressings to apply.

FRACTURES, BREAKS & SPRAINS

Broken Bones & Fractures
Symptoms

Sharp pain and tenderness near the injury, swelling; Loss of function of the injured part; Deformity or unnatural movement of part at fracture site; Impaired circulation resulting in numbness, tingling and a pale or bluish skin tone.

Action

1. Support the injured part until fracture is immobilized.
2. Immobilize fracture in position found. Protect the injured part in soft padding (may be improvised from blankets, jackets, plastic or leafy vegetation). Bandage the broken part to the body or prepare a splint.
3. Slings may be improvised from bandana, belt, shirt, pants, blanket or any available non-stretching piece of cloth.
4. Splints can be improvised from sticks, boards, tree limbs or cardboard. Either place one splint on each side of fracture and tie the splints together with bandages or tie the fractured bone to a board. Bandages may be improvised from belts, handkerchiefs or ripped pieces of cloth.
5. Monitor for shock and transport for medical help as soon as possible.

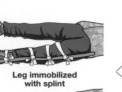

Leg immobilized with splint

Triangular Bandana

Leg immobilized with other leg

Sprains or Dislocated Joints
Symptoms

Sharp pain and tenderness near the injury; Swelling; Loss of range of motion or inability to use joint.

Action

1. Avoid putting pressure on injured limb/area.
2. Bind injury to reduce swelling and support limb.

Ankle immobilized with blanket

CHECKING CIRCULATION

After bandaging a limb, check for circulation every 10 minutes. Press finger or toenail until it turns pale, then release; color should return quickly. If it does not, the bandage is too tight and should be reapplied.

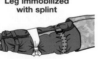

EYE INJURY

Common injuries include cut/torn eyelids, cut/scratched eyeball, extruded eyeball (out of socket) or burns to eye.

1. In all cases, help victim to lie on their back and be still and not move their eyes.
2. If an object becomes embedded in the eye, place the cleanest available dressing over the injured eye(s) but DO NOT put pressure on the eyeball(s). Cover embedded object so there is no pressure on the object. Always bandage both eyes since eyes move together and this will lessen the chance of damage to the injured eye.

Bandage both eyes.   **Cover embedded objects.**

POISONING

Usually occurs when poisons are ingested. The treatment varies depending upon the type and volume of poison swallowed.

1. Seek medical help immediately.
2. If victim is conscious, wipe out or rinse mouth of any remaining poison.
3. Do not induce vomiting or drink fluids to dilute the poison.
4. Determine what poison has been ingested.
5. Monitor breathing and be prepared to treat for shock.

DIARRHEA AND VOMITING

Diarrhea and vomiting can be caused by many conditions including stress. The most common causes in a wilderness situation are contamination from handling unclean food waste or drinking unpurified water. Common back-country diseases like giardia cause vomiting and diarrhea which in turn cause dehydration and can be fatal. It is critical to rehydrate with fresh, uncontaminated water. Suspect water should be disinfected by boiling for at least five minutes or treated with purification tablets.

SURVIVAL KIT RESOURCES

Your survival kit includes the basics that you will need to administer self aid in most circumstances:

Bandana – is useful to protect sunburned areas, as a sling, as dressing for a wound and, if needed, as a tourniquet.

Paracord/bank line – cordage can be used to bind dressings or hold splints in place, bank line can be used for sutures if necessary.

Needle – can be heated/sterilized to do fine sliver removal and to suture severe wounds.

Duct tape – bandaid for cuts, lashing for splints, wrap for sprains, mending material for hats and clothing.

Water purification tablets – clean water will help avoid illness, and is essential to help rehydrate if injured or ill.

BITES & STINGS

If you are injured by an animal, in all cases, seek medical treatment at the earliest possible time.

Flying Insects – Bites & Stings

The best tactic for self-protection is avoidance. Avoid areas where bees are feeding on flowers if you can. Meat-eating hornets are attracted to strong smells and brightly colored clothing, so beware.

If you are attacked by bees or hornets, run away from the swarm and seek shelter if you can find it. If you are being stung, cover your eyes, nose and mouth with your arms or a piece of clothing. Do not flail your arms or attack the bees – especially killer bees – as this will cause them to intensify their attack.

If you are stung by bees, try to remove the stingers as soon as possible by stroking them out with your knife blade or fingernail. Don't squeeze the poison sac at the end of the stinger as this will release more venom.

Honey Bee
Can sting only once and leaves barbed stinger and poison sac attached to victim.

Hornet
Can sting repeatedly.

Ticks

Disease-carrying bugs found in brushy areas jump on passing animals, including humans, and migrate to insulated areas in the head, armpit and groin. Check for ticks daily and remove by applying slow pressure. Get whole insect out. Do not burn with a match. Clean wound thoroughly.

Actual Size
Wood Tick

Snakes

The bite from a poisonous snake usually causes a burning sensation in the affected area, followed by swelling and discoloration. Most venomous snakes inject venom deeply. It is not advisable to cut the wound and try to suck out the poison since this will only cause the venom to spread more quickly into the bloodstream. Following a bite, the primary concern is to slow blood flow between the bite area and the heart. Try to relax (if you are the victim), in order to slow your heart rate. Immobilize the affected limb (use a splint if you can) at a level below the heart. Wash the wound if you can.

Rattlesnake

Mammals

The main danger from mammal bites is the risk of infection from tetanus or rabies. While almost any wild animal can have rabies, the most common carriers in North America are bats, raccoons, foxes and coyotes. Rabies is usually transmitted by a bite or scratch. If bitten by a potentially rabid animal, let the wound bleed to help cleanse it, then thoroughly wash it.

Bears, moose, elk and large cats are dangerous to humans. Avoid carcasses and putrid smelling areas (or approach very carefully) – these could be bear food caches. Be aware of moose and elk in rut season – a bull will charge without provocation if you find yourself in their territory. Mountain lions and other wild cats are generally reclusive, but can attack humans, especially small children.

Raccoon

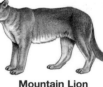

Mountain Lion